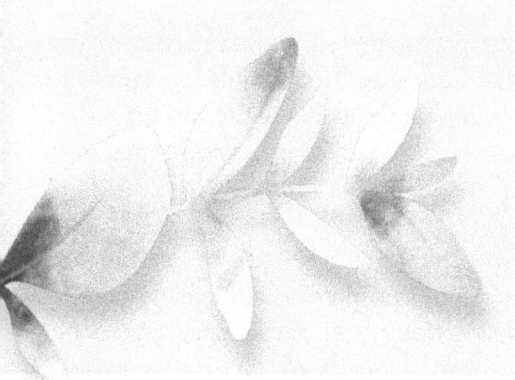

Breakthrough Toolbook

If I Can Heal, You Can Heal

WRITTEN BY

Delfina Geus

T he breakthrough tools in this booklet will help you access the richness of freedom available to you with Jesus. The power of each of these breakthrough tools is found in him and nowhere else. The power is not in the words written on this paper and it's not in the ritual or routine of the prayer. The healing power is Jesus himself. He will heal you by pulling out all of the stubborn weeds that have grown over the good seeds in your heart. Then, he will reveal truth to you so that you can know who you really are and step into your set-free future.

Deliverance has nothing to do with your past. It has everything to do with your future and getting rid of the obstacles that have stood in your way. This book is for dreamers, believers, fighters, and survivors who are tired of waking up to a reality less than what they know they were designed for, for those who are ready to step into all what they were made for.

This is not a self-help book. There are no recipes, remedies, quick-tips, secrets or how-to's in this book. It's a book of miracles and believing in the more of God, that the more of God will establish you in freedom in your right life. Nothing about your past can change the future God has for you. Your future is untouched by trauma. Who you are has existed in God's mind long before you experienced pain. The darkest day of your story can't take away from what God has planned for you.

If I can heal, you can heal

Dedication

This book is dedicated to
those of you who still believe in miracles
(and to those of you who wish you still believed.)

Blessings & Prayers

My Opening Prayer for You
"Jesus, thank you so much that you're already here. Thank you that you are next to each and every person reading this book right now. You knew this day would come. It's a divine appointment that was written in your book of life from the beginning of time. Make the words of this book personal to them. Lead them into the miracles hidden in the pages of this book. Help them believe that what you did for me, you will do for them. I ask you Jesus to make your presence known even more, right now wherever each reader finds themselves, so that they will know that you're with them and closer than ever before. Make your presence known, and lead their spirits into the greatest freedom they've ever known."

Coming to Jesus & Asking Him to Rewrite Your Past
"Jesus, I'm ready to try things your way. I want you to come into my life and change everything. I don't care about my past anymore. I want you to rewrite it and heal every impossible thing about my life. Show me that you are God!"

Letting Go of False Support Systems
"Jesus, this is really difficult and scary for me to do, but I am trusting that you'll have my back. I surrender, right now, all the things, habits, people, thoughts and emotions I've been turning to for comfort, and I turn to you instead. I ask you to be my strength and fill me with true power so that I can live the life you designed for me from the beginning."

Fully Surrendering Counterfeit Comforts
"Jesus, I give you all of my counterfeit support systems. I'm sorry for all the times I didn't reach for you or lean on you when I was in pain. I want to lean on you fully now. Please heal me from every wound, every scar and every demon that has kept me from living my best life with you. Reorder every part of me that's out of order so that I can build a strong and powerful life with you and feel contained and safe in your comfort."

Asking Jesus to Increase Your Faith
"Jesus, I ask you to increase my faith. Help me to imagine a future without pain. Show me what you have planned for me for my life. I want to know that I'm not too late to do the things my heart desires to do. Send me a confirmation. Give me visions, dreams and encounters with people that speak your words powerfully to me about my future. I want to dream with you, Lord. Help me believe!"

Scriptural Declarations

I have authority to trample every spirit of darkness!

Luke 10:18-20 (TPT) "Jesus replied, "While you were ministering, I watched Satan topple until he fell suddenly from heaven like lightning to the ground. Now you understand that I have imparted to you my authority to trample over his kingdom. You will trample upon every demon before you and overcome every power Satan possesses. Absolutely nothing will harm you as you walk in this authority. However, your real source of joy isn't merely that these spirits submit to your authority, but that your names are written in the journals of heaven and that you belong to God's kingdom. This is the true source of your authority."

No weapon formed against me will prosper!

Isaiah 54:17 (NLT) "But in that coming day no weapon turned against you will succeed. You will silence every voice raised up to accuse you. These benefits are enjoyed by the servants of the LORD; their vindication will come from me. I, the LORD, have spoken!"

He who is in me (God) is greater than he (the devil) who is in the world.

1 John 4:4 (NLT) "But you belong to God, my dear children. You have already won a victory over those people, because the Spirit who lives in you is greater than the spirit who lives in the world."

God has not given me a spirit of fear, but a spirit of love, power and a sound mind.

2 Timothy 1:7 (KJV) "For God hath not given us the spirit of fear; but of power, and of love, and of a sound mind."

Who the son sets free, is free indeed!

John 8:36 (NLT) "So if the Son sets you free, you are truly free."

I am a new creation. The old is gone, the new has come.

2 Corinthians 5:17 (NLT), "This means that anyone who belongs to Christ has become a new person. The old life is gone; a new life has begun!"

BREAKTHROUGH TOOLS for your

POWER ENCOUNTER WITH GOD

DISCERNMENT GUIDE
UNDERSTANDING THE INFORMATION YOU'RE RECEIVING

TAKING THOUGHTS CAPTIVE
NAILING THOUGHTS & SPIRITUAL INFLUENCES TO THE CROSS

REBUKING DEMONIC SPIRITS
SENDING AWAY SPIRITUAL INFLUENCES, ATMOSPHERES & ATTACKS

INTERVIEWING STRONG EMOTIONS
BREAKING AGREEMENTS WITH DEMONS AND STRONG EMOTIONS

EMOTIONS LIST
A LIST TO HELP YOU KNOW WHAT YOU'RE FEELING IN YOUR SPIRIT AND SOUL

FORGIVENESS ENCOUNTER
CLOSING DOORS OF TORMENT BY RELEASING FORGIVENESS

BREAKING GENERATIONAL CURSES
CANCELING FAMILY CURSES & CLAIMING GENERATIONAL BLESSINGS

BREAKING WORD CURSES & VOWS
BREAKING AGREEMENTS WITH GENERAL CURSES & SPIRITUAL CONTRACTS

BREAKING SOULTIES
RELEASING BAGGAGE FROM SPIRITUAL & NATURAL ATTACHMENTS

DISCERNMENT GUIDE

UNDERSTANDING THE INFORMATION YOU'RE RECEIVING

Information comes at you about past, present or future situations in the form of:

| Feeling or sensing something | Knowing or thinking something | Having a physical sensation |

Talk to the Holy Spirit about it.

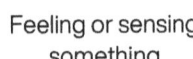

"*Holy Spirit, what is happening?*"

Connection with God

• You're feeling God's spirit, which manifests in all kinds of beautiful ways (ie: miracles, signs and wonders, goosebumps, etc.)

• You are experiencing the fruit of the spirit: love, joy, peace, forbearance, kindness, goodness, faithfulness, gentleness and self-control. (Galatians 5:22-26)

• Your mind is consumed with thoughts of heaven: all things good, noble, right, true pure. (Philippians 4:8)

• You're having a revelation or vision or trance where God is showing you things from his perspective and you're left with awe and wonder and good surprise.

(*The page does not fit all the endless possibilities of how God talks.)

Spiritual things

• You're picking up on a spiritual atmosphere
• You're picking up on someone else's stuff in the spirit
• The enemy is trying to make you think you're not set free by having old things manifest in your mind, desires or emotions

Natural things

• You have a need or boundary and you need to eat, speak, ask, rest, do, etc.

• **God is touching a pain-point or trigger and it feels demonic, but it's actually God pulling something out of you in order to heal it, which is causing you to have emotions, thoughts or physical sensations that feel like demonic attacks.**

DISCERNMENT GUIDE

UNDERSTANDING THE INFORMATION YOU'RE RECEIVING

③ Ask the Holy Spirit what to do.

" Holy Spirit, what do I do?"

In response to a demonic attack, listen to what God is saying to do. Some things I do include worshiping, praying, declaring scriptures out loud, taking communion, doing a prophetic act, breaking agreements with lies, rebuking devils, dancing, singing, creating and reading the Bible. Other times, I just laugh and move on with my day without giving the enemy much attention. The Holy Spirit knows how to guide you through every situation. Ask him what to do.

Healing with God: Listen to what God is saying to do. He might lead you into using one of these tools for breakthrough:

- Breaking agreements with lies
- Breaking generational curses
- Rebuking spirits
- Breaking soul ties
- Forgiveness encounter

(*These tools are explained in the following few pages.)

Remember: When the Holy Spirit gets ready to free you from something, all of hell might break loose. You are not going crazy when this happens, there is nothing wrong with you, and you're not alone. Keep your eyes on Jesus. Listen to his voice. Follow the instructions of the Holy Spirit. God has a plan to free you from bondage, even when and especially if it seems like things get worse before they get better. God has not abandoned you. Stand firm!

A note about processing endlessly: When God starts talking about something, it's because he's ready to heal you right then and there. Healing with God doesn't take forever, and after he's healed you, he doesn't go back into your pain. After you've dealt with your pain with Jesus and the topic gets brought up to your attention over and over again, it's probably not God talking. The enemy loves to keep us perpetually 'figuring things out' in our pain and in our past, when deliverance is actually about being brought out of our past and out of our pain into a set-free present and future. If you're feeling stuck in an endless loop of introspection, fear or 'healing and feeling' mode, ask the Holy Spirit what's happening. Then, possibly, rebuke the spirit of trauma.

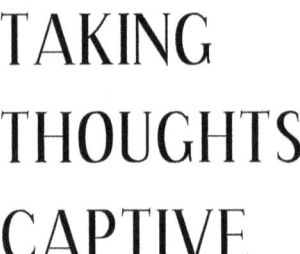

TAKING THOUGHTS CAPTIVE

NAILING THOUGHTS & SPIRITUAL INFLUENCES TO THE CROSS

1 – When you sense that you've picked up a lie or something from the enemy in your spirit, ask the Holy Spirit for discernment:
- "Holy Spirit, what lie am I believing?"
- "Holy Spirit, what's coming against me?"
- "Holy Spirit, what's the root of this emotion, thought or desire?"

2 – Once you identify the lies and spirits coming against you, give them to Jesus by saying:
- "I nail _____ to the cross and break all agreements I've made with it."

3 – Ask Jesus what truth he has in exchange for this lie and listen to what the Holy Spirit tells you:
- "Jesus, what truth do you want to give me in exchange for this?"

> "He canceled the record of the charges against us and took it away by nailing it to the cross. In this way, he disarmed the spiritual rulers and authorities. He shamed them publicly by his victory over them on the cross."
> **Colossians 2:14-15 (NLT)**

REBUKING DEMONIC SPIRITS

SENDING AWAY SPIRITUAL INFLUENCES, ATMOSPHERES AND ATTACKS

When you sense a demonic spirit or demonic spiritual atmosphere coming against you, you can stand in your authority in Jesus and command it to leave by saying:
- "Spirit of _____ get out, in Jesus name!"
- "I command this atmosphere to shift now in the name of Jesus."

If you feel like you've come into agreement with this spiritual atmosphere or demonic spirit in any way, break agreements with it as well.

If you're facing a strong attack that persists, continue to resist it and turn to Jesus through an active display of faith, like:
- **Making declarations of scriptures out loud**
- **Turning on worship music and worshiping God boldly**
- **Taking communion**
- **Prophetically putting on the armor of Christ**
- **Or, if the Holy Spirit says to radically ignore the enemy, then radically ignore the enemy!**

> "I have given you authority to trample on snakes and scorpions and to overcome all the power of the enemy; nothing will harm you."
> **Luke 10:19 (NIV)**

INTERVIEWING STRONG EMOTIONS

EXCHANGING STRONG EMOTIONS & INFLUENCES FOR GOD'S LOVE

1 - Ask the Holy Spirit what contract you've made with the strong emotion or spiritual influence you're picking up on in your spirit. Ask the Holy Spirit to show you what counterfeit comfort or benefit it was giving to you:

- "Holy Spirit, what does ____spirit/emotion____ do for me?"

2 - Listen to what the Holy Spirit has to say. Once you learn why what that emotion or spiritual influence was doing for you, release it back to Jesus and ask him to replace it with something good and heavenly:

- "Jesus, I give you ____spirit/emotion____ and all it does for me. What do you have in exchange for me?"

> "You perceive every movement of my heart and soul, and you understand my every thought before it even enters my mind."
> **Psalms 139:2 (TPT)**

EMOTIONS LIST

A LIST TO HELP YOU KNOW WHAT YOU'RE FEELING IN YOUR SPIRIT AND SOUL

ANGER
Angry
Annoyed
Irritated
Frustrated
Enraged
Bitter
Resentful
Stubborn
Rigid
Tense

FEAR
Afraid
Worried
Concerned
Scared
Terrified
Spooked
On alert
Anxious
Insecure
Nervous
Paranoid
Dreading
Resistant
Unsettled
Unsure
On guard
Frozen
Frantic

SADNESS
Sad
Down
Depressed
Hopeless
Disappointed
Defeated
Let down
Regretful
Despairing
Misunderstood
Grieved
Longing
Heavy
Slow

SURPRISE
Surprised
Shocked
In awe
Caught off guard
Not ready

SHAME
Shameful
Embarrassed
Unworthy
Unspecial
Unloved

PAIN
Hurt
Crushed
Lonely
Betrayed
Weary
In pain
Broken
Disconnected
Broken-hearted
Rejected
Unwanted
Aching
Anguished

DISGUST
Disgusted
Repulsed by
Offended
Grossed out
Disinterested

GUILT
Guilty
Bad
Convicted
Blamed
At fault
Condemned
Remorseful

PLEASURE/JOY
Happy
Joyful
Excited
Interested
Drawn to
Enjoying
Anticipating
Eager
Fulfilled
Understood
Connected
Accepted
Worthy
Peaceful
Relaxed
Expectant
Hopeful
Proud
Radiant
Seen
Loved
Loving
Energized
Confident
Ready
Willing
Trusting
Strong
Free

FORGIVENESS ENCOUNTER

CLOSING DOORS OF DEMONIC TORMENT BY RELEASING FORGIVENESS

Ask the Holy Spirit to show you who he wants you to release forgiveness to, then go through this forgiveness encounter:

1 - Picture Jesus standing in front of you next to the person you're forgiving. Give Jesus any strong emotion that comes up, by saying:

- "Jesus, I'm feeling _____. I need you to comfort me."

2 - Speak forgiveness directly to the person for all the things that they did to hurt you, like this:

- "__(Name of person)__ I forgive you for _____."

3 - Go deeper. Ask the Holy Spirit to show you the consequences of what that person did. This would include every physical, emotional, mental and spiritual injury that this person caused you. Release forgiveness to them for each and every one of those things:

- "I forgive you for causing me to feel / think / do

4 - Release this person back to Jesus. Ask Jesus to bless the person, and then ask Jesus to close every door of torment:

- "Jesus, I choose to forgive _____ and I release them back to you. I ask that you bless them with _____ . Please close every door of torment that I opened with my unforgiveness.

FORGIVENESS ENCOUNTER

CLOSING DOORS OF DEMONIC TORMENT BY RELEASING FORGIVENESS

Example of the forgiveness encounter:

"Dad, I forgive you for beating me and leaving bruises all over my body. I forgive you for the shame this caused me when I had to go to school and my friends asked about it. I forgive you for how this opened the door to fear every time I was at home. I forgive you for how your actions shaped the way I see men and people in authority. I forgive you for denying the pain you caused me and for not being sorry. I forgive you for making me so mad and for bringing so much anger into my life and all my relationships. I forgive you for teaching me that violence is okay, and for how that got me into so much trouble in my life. I forgive you for being a terrible father and making me feel worthless and broken.

"Jesus, I give my dad back to you, and all the pain and hurt he caused me, I give it to you now too. I ask you to close every door of torment that I opened by holding onto this bitterness and pain for so long. I choose to forgive my dad, and I release him back to you now, Jesus. I ask that you would bless my dad to find help and to encounter you."

You can revisit this tool as often as the Holy Spirit prompts you to do so with different people in your life. You can forgive anyone, even the people who are no longer in your life and those who are no longer living. The prayer is between you and God.

> "And whenever you stand praying, if you find that you carry something in your heart against another person, release him and forgive him so that your Father in heaven will also release you and forgive you of your faults."
> **Mark 11:25 (TPT)**

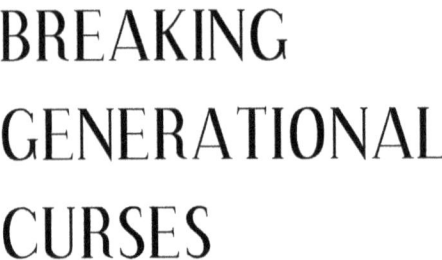

BREAKING GENERATIONAL CURSES

CANCELING FAMILY CURSES & CLAIMING GENERATIONAL BLESSINGS

Once the Holy Spirit has helped you identify which family curses he wants to break, say this prayer:

"Jesus, I ask in your name that you break the power of _____ which has manifested in my family as a generational curse. I ask you to replace every cursed habit and pattern that has come from this generational curse and replace it with a supernatural generational blessing by the power of your cross. Lord, what generational blessings do you have in exchange for this curse?"

Listen to what Jesus has for your family line in exchange for these curses.

> "I will certainly bless you. I will multiply your descendants beyond number, like the stars in the sky and the sand on the seashore. Your descendants will conquer the cities of their enemies."
> **Genesis 22:17 (NLT)**

BREAKING WORD CURSES & VOWS

BREAKING AGREEMENTS
WITH GENERAL CURSES &
SPIRITUAL CONTRACTS

1 - Ask the Holy Spirit to show you the word curse he wants to break off of your life. Then pray:

"In Jesus name, I break all agreements I've made with the word curse _____ . I ask you Jesus to send the demonic power of these words out of my life, out of my thoughts, out of my emotions and out of my desires and behaviors. Lord, set a guard in my spirit so I never partner with this word curse again."

2 - Ask Jesus if there are any vows you've made in response to the word curse, then break agreements with them:
- "Holy Spirit, are there vows I've made in response to this word curse?"
- "In Jesus name, I break all agreements I've made with this vow. I ask you Jesus to break the power of this vow off of my life."

3 - Then ask Jesus what truth he wants to give you in exchange for that lie:
- "Jesus, what's the truth about how you see me?"

You can use the words Jesus speaks to you to make powerful declarations about yourself anytime the enemy or someone else tries to introduce these word curses and lies to you in the future.

> "But in that coming day no weapon turned against you will succeed. You will silence every voice raised up to accuse you. These benefits are enjoyed by the servants of the LORD; their vindication will come from me. I, the LORD, have spoken!" **Isaiah 54:17 (NLT)**

BREAKING SOUL TIES

RELEASING BAGGAGE FROM SPIRITUAL AND NATURAL ATTACHMENTS

Ask the Holy Spirit to show you where you have made ungodly soul ties with any person, place, thing or substance. Then pray this prayer:

"In the name of Jesus, I ask you God to break every ungodly soul tie I've made with _____. I ask you to cancel out every exchange I made with _____. Take out of me anything ungodly that I received from them, and I pray you would remove from them anything ungodly I gave to them. I ask you to speak your healing words of peace and comfort into my soul and spirit to fill the place where this ungodly soul tie existed. God, what's the truth you want me to know about this relationship?

Listen to the truth God has for you about the relationship.

> "For the word of God is alive and powerful. It is sharper than the sharpest two-edged sword, cutting between soul and spirit, between joint and marrow. It exposes our innermost thoughts and desires. Nothing in all creation is hidden from God. Everything is naked and exposed before his eyes, and he is the one to whom we are accountable."
> **Hebrews 4:12-13 (NLT)**

Notes:

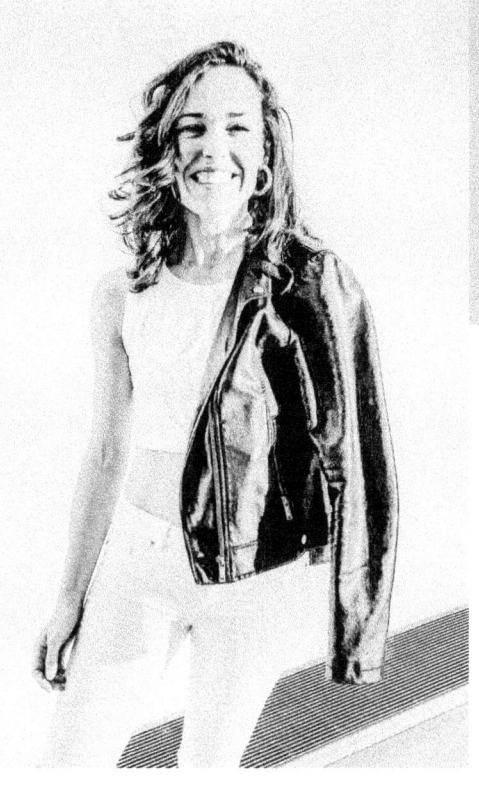

About the author

Delfina Geus is a singer/songwriter and entrepreneur from Los Angeles, CA.

www.delfinageus.com

Have a testimony?

I would love to hear from you! Send me a letter about what God did for you at:

Delfina Geus
P.O. Box 70411
Project City, CA 96079
United States of America

Thank you!

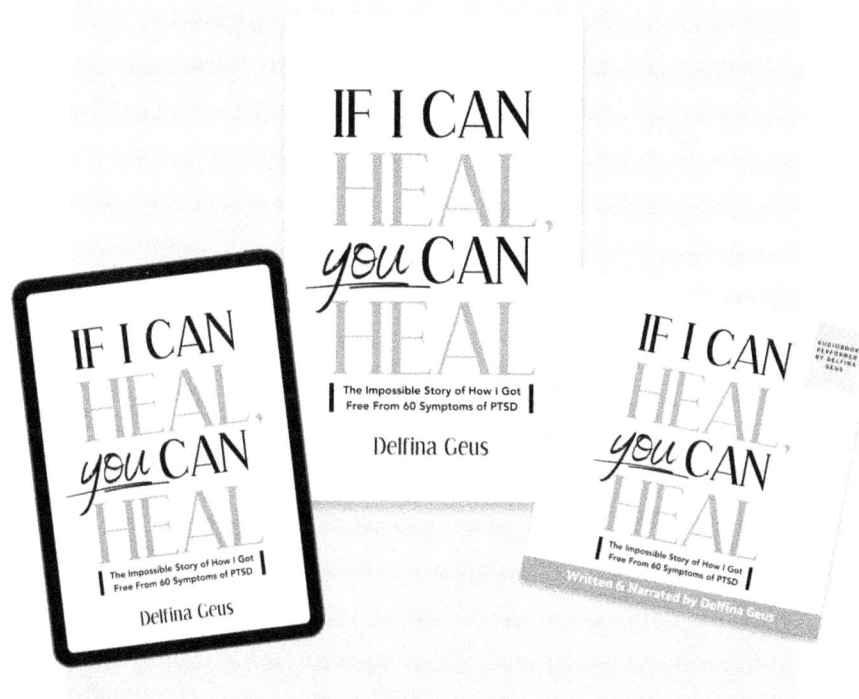

This title is available on Amazon in paperback, e-book and audiobook

in Deutsch, Español and Français

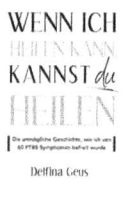
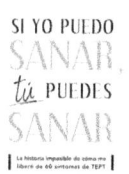
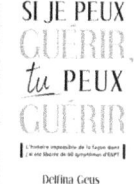

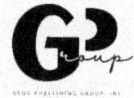

Copyright & Permissions

If I Can Heal, You Can Heal: Breakthrough Toolbook
by Delfina Geus. Copyright © 2023 by Delfina Entertainment, LLC. All Rights Reserved.

Content may be quoted or printed on paper and distributed free of charge for personal use, religious and college classes, and study guides so long as no changes are made and proper credit is given to the author. No part of this manuscript may be used or reproduced in any matter whatsoever for commercial use or resale purposes without prior written permission from the publisher, except in the case of brief quotations embodied in critical articles and reviews and certain other noncommercial uses permitted by copyright law. For more information please contact: permissions@geuspublishing.com

Scripture quotations marked (NIV) are taken from the Holy Bible, New International Version®, NIV®. Copyright © 1973, 1978, 1984, 2011 by Biblica, Inc.™ Used by permission of Zondervan. All rights reserved worldwide. www.zondervan.com. The "NIV" and "New International Version" are trademarks registered in the United States Patent and Trademark Office by Biblica, Inc.™ Scripture quotations marked (TPT) are from The Passion Translation®. Copyright © 2017, 2018, 2020 by Passion & Fire Ministries, Inc. Used by permission. All rights reserved. ThePassionTranslation.com. Scripture quotations marked (NASB) are taken from the (NASB®) New American Standard Bible®, Copyright © 1960, 1971, 1977, 1995, 2020 by The Lockman Foundation. Used by permission. All rights reserved. Lockman.org Scripture quotations marked (NLT) are taken from the Holy Bible, New Living Translation, copyright ©1996, 2004, 2015 by Tyndale House Foundation. Used by permission of Tyndale House Publishers, Carol Stream, Illinois 60188. All rights reserved. Scripture quotations marked (KJV) are taken from The Authorized (King James) Version. Rights in the Authorized Version in the United Kingdom are vested in the Crown. Reproduced by permission of the Crown's patentee, Cambridge University Press. Scripture quotations taken from the Amplified® Bible (AMP), Copyright © 2015 by The Lockman Foundation. Used by permission. Lockman.org

Geus Publishing Group, Inc.
P.O. Box 70411
Project City, CA 96079
United States of America

ISBN: 979-8-9895662-9-7 (paperback)

FIRST EDITION 2023
For Worldwide Distribution, Printed in the United States
www.delfinageus.com

www.ingramcontent.com/pod-product-compliance
Lightning Source LLC
Chambersburg PA
CBHW070755050426
42449CB00010B/2489